Life is a Wiggle:
Dance Like a Sea Animal – Level I

Published by The Whole Works® New York

Written by: Ettie Steg and Monika Pia
Cover and book design: Ettie Steg and Monika Pia
Dance, choreography, video production and its stills: Ettie Steg
Graphics and dance-path illustrations: Ettie Steg
Sea creature illustrations and cover photo: Monika Pia

Dancer and voice-over: Jaylene Rodriguez O'Garro
Sound design – Sea Waves: Hajime Aoki

Disclaimer: While the publisher and authors have used their best efforts in preparing this book and its video, they make no representations or warranties as to the accuracy or completeness of the information and specifically disclaim any implied fitness for a particular purpose or for a particular person. The advice and exercises shown may not be suitable for your physicality. Always consult a qualified medical professional before beginning any exercise program. Warm up well, before exercising, and cool down afterwards.

Ettie Steg
Visit her web site at www.DanceForMyLife.com and read her articles about dance at SelfGrowth.com

Monika Pia
Visit her web site at www.ComeToLifeWithBooks.com

Produced in the United States of America.

ISBN: 978-0-692-00713-6

Life is a Wiggle

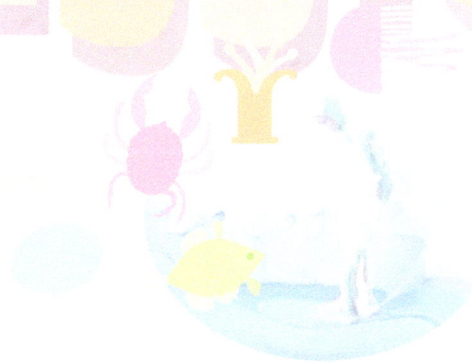

The joyful energy of constantly-moving sea animals inspired us to create for you, your child, and the child within you, this childrens' introduction to dance.

As a bonus we include a delightful three-minute video performed by Jaylene, who is eight. Dance along with her as she describes how to bring each unique sea animal in these pages to life.

We hope you enjoy doing these movements to enrich your lives and stir your imagination.

Contents
Part 1: Basic moves
Always warm up gently before exercising and cool down afterwards by walking slowly around

Download the video at
TheWholeWorksDownload.com
Also sign up there for your free e-mail dance tips

Every sea animal has its own wiggle
Wiggle wiggle wiggle

- Let's wiggle like a fish — 1
- Let's wiggle like a crab — 2
- Let's wiggle like a turtle — 3
- Let's wiggle like a coral polyp — 4
- Let's wiggle like a jelly fish — 5

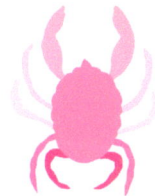

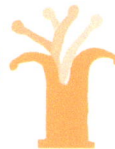

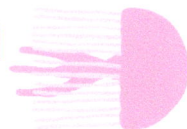

Contents
Part 2: Moving on

Remember your warm-up and cool-down

Now keep on wiggling and expand what we've learned

- **Let's join the five wiggles**   6

- **Add the fantastic**   7

- **Create your own creature**   8-9

- **And travel new paths**   10-14

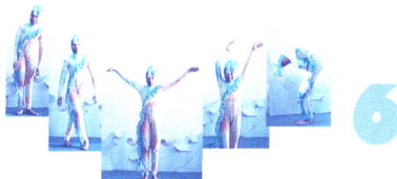

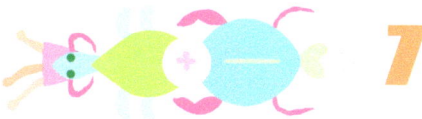

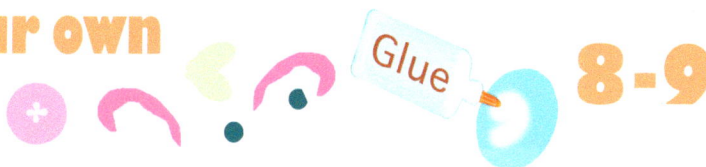

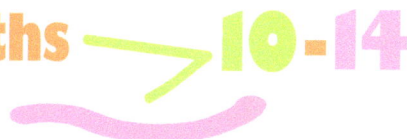

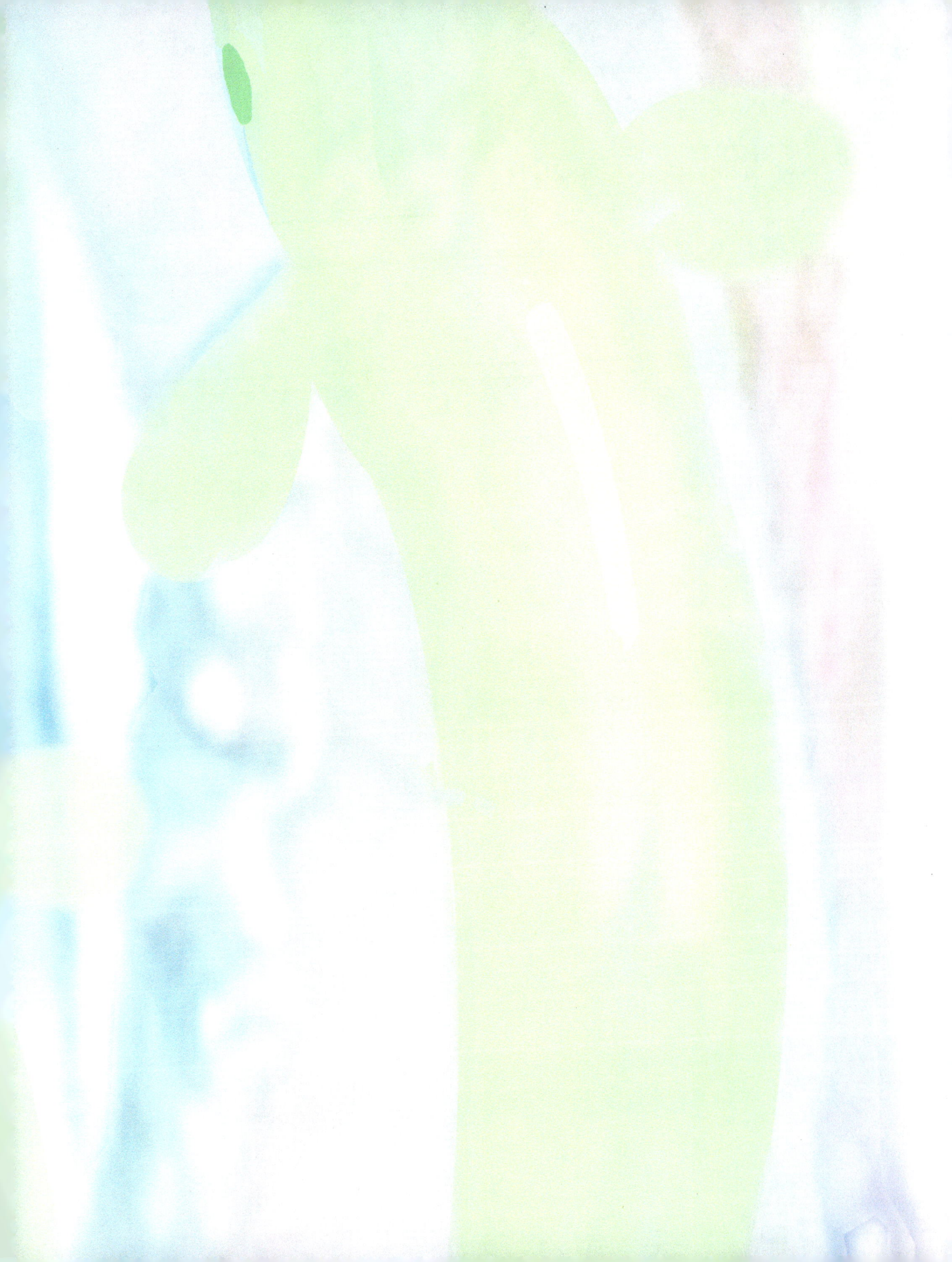

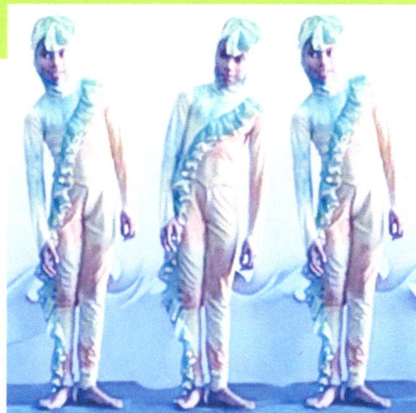

When the **fish** swims, it curves its spine from side to side. Stand tall and bend yourself from side to side.

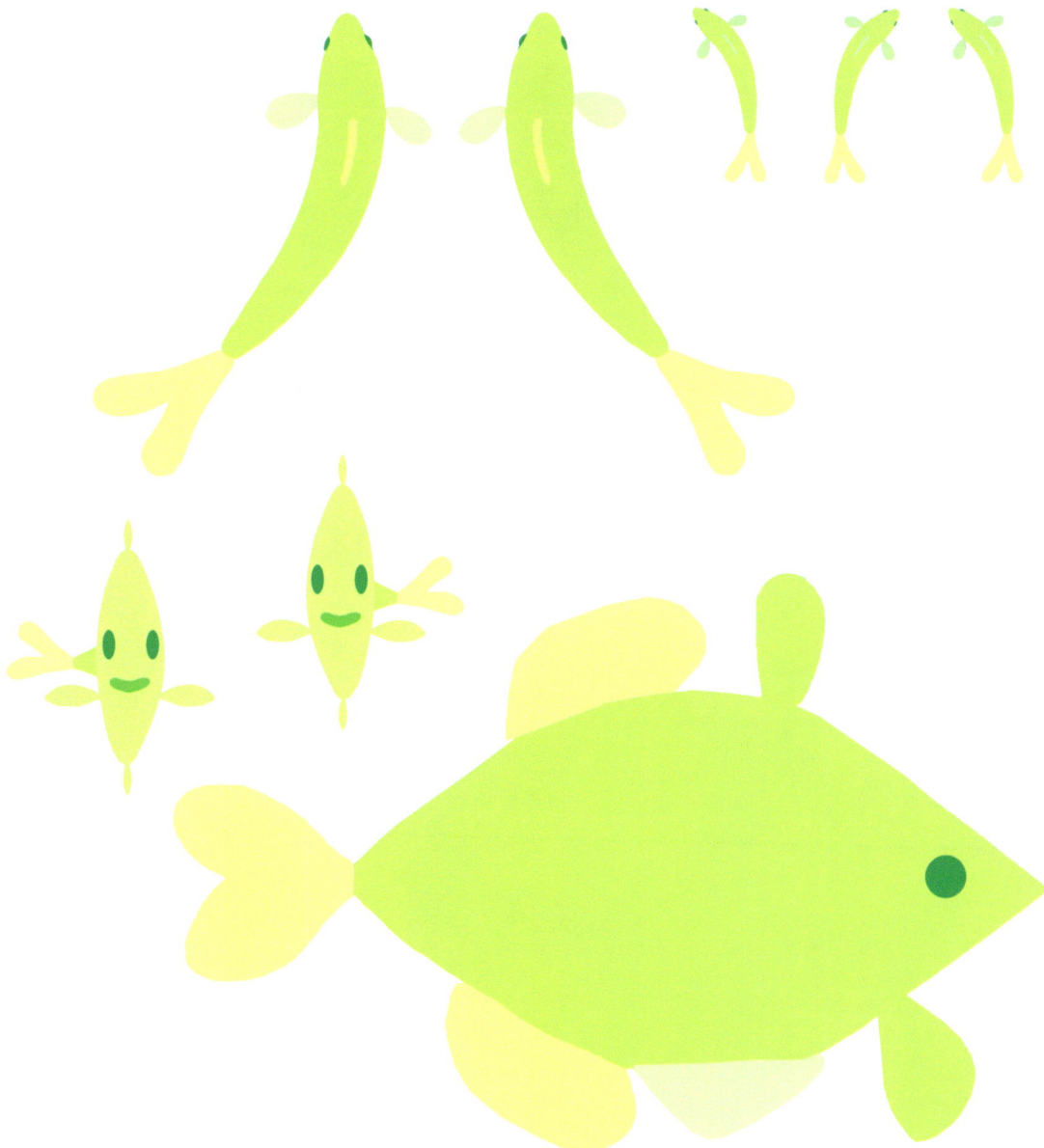

The **crab** walks sideways by criss-crossing its legs.

Cross one leg to the front and stand on it. Move your back leg sideways in the same direction.

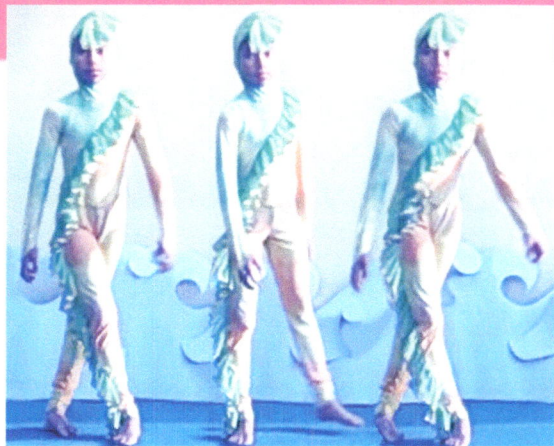

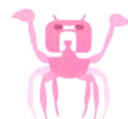

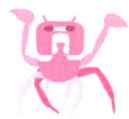

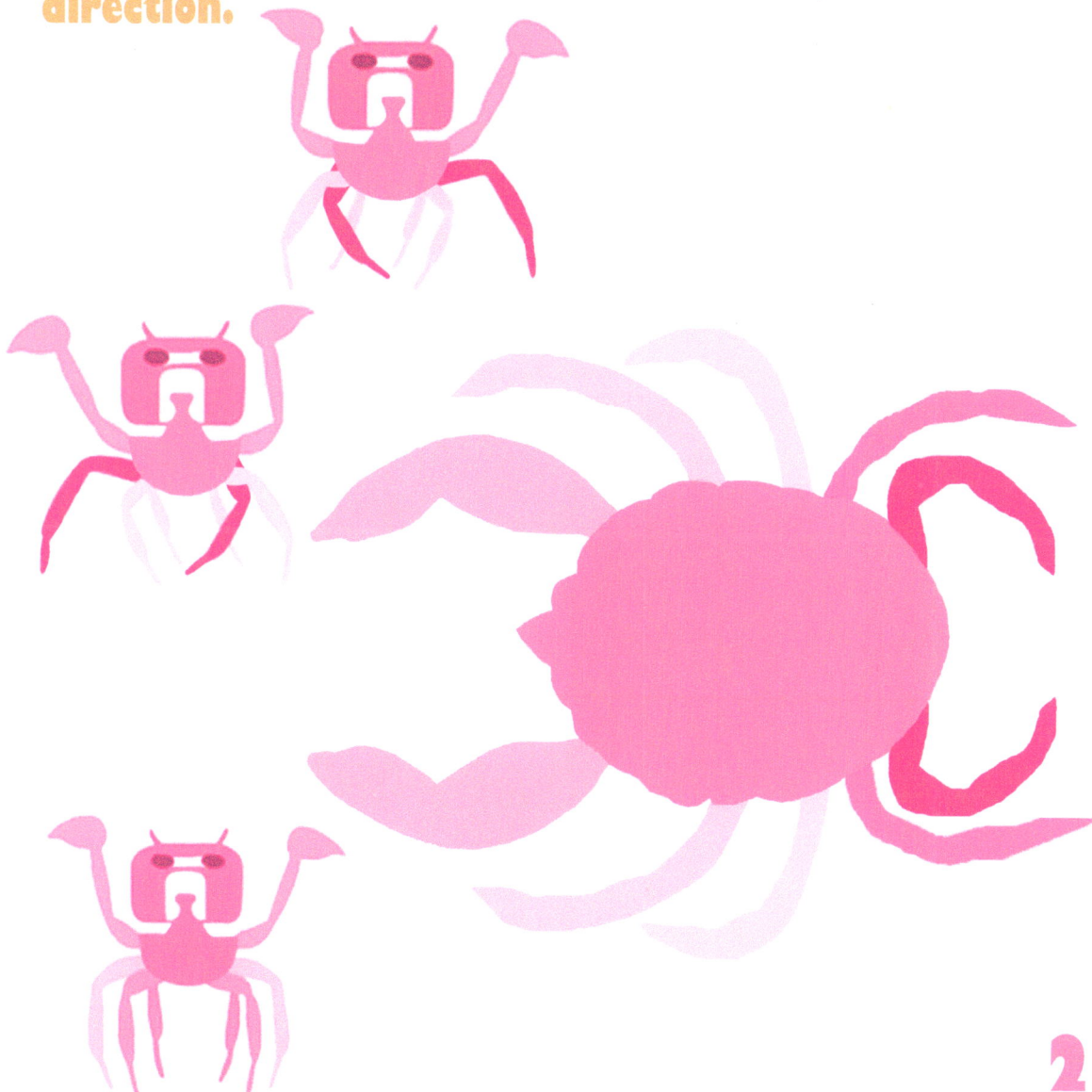

2

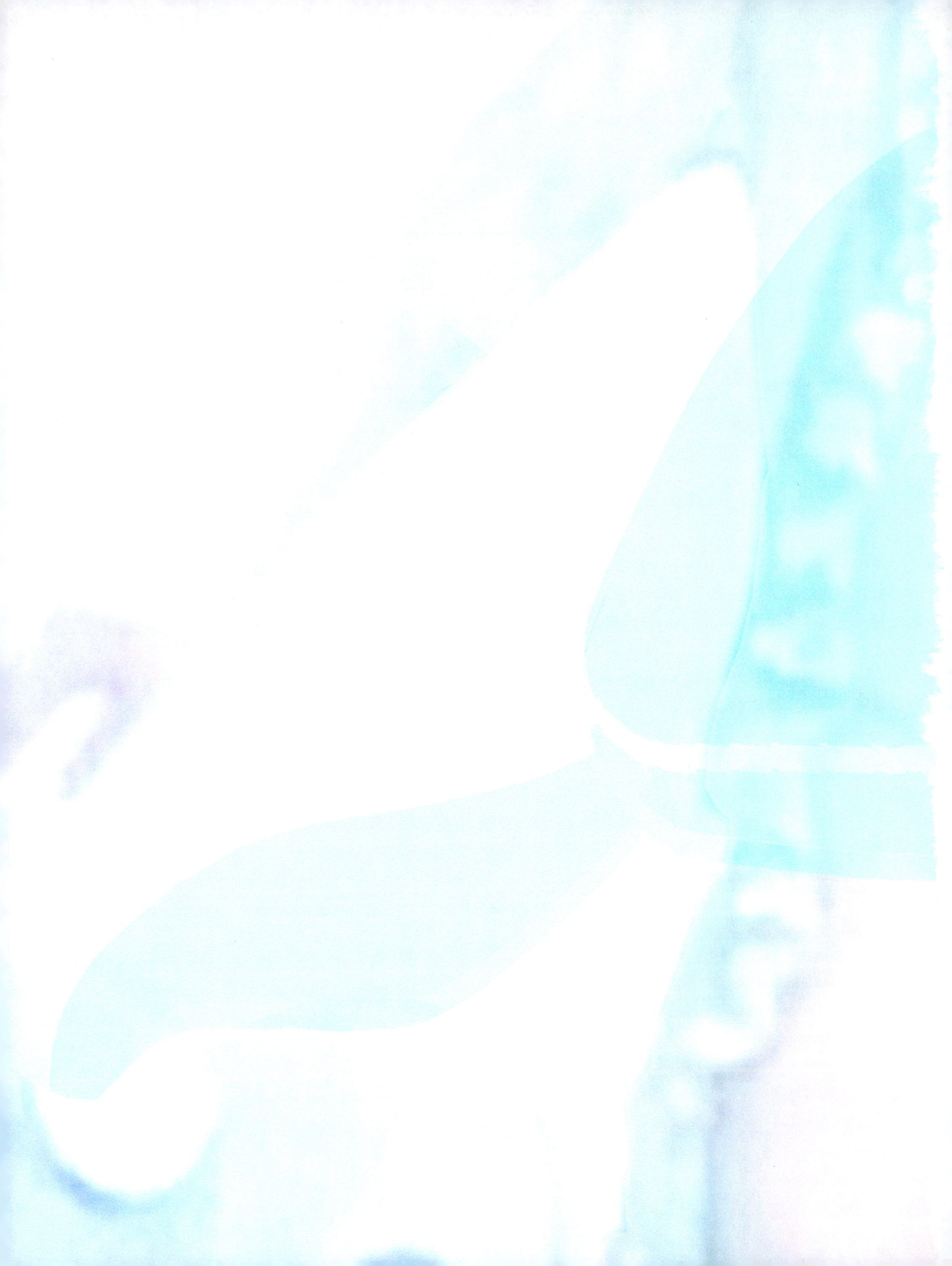

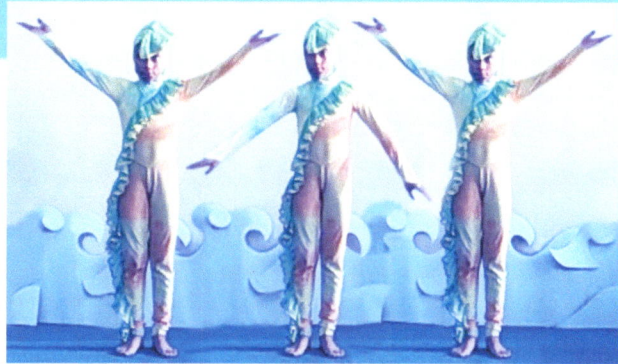

The **turtle** moves its front fins like a bird moves its wings.

Reach your arms to the side and move them up and down in a figure eight.

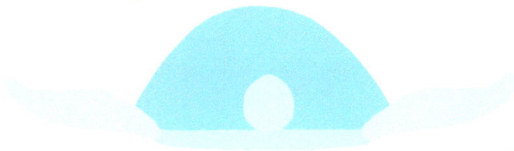

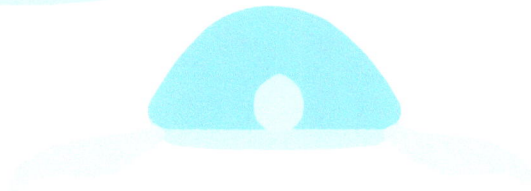

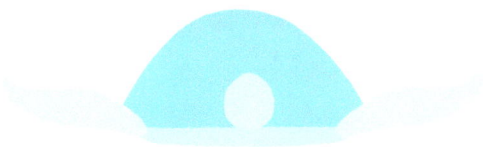

3

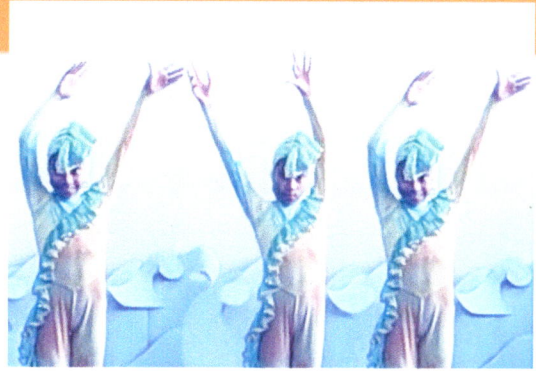

The **coral polyp** moves its tentacles to feed itself.

Kneel down, reach and sway your arms and fingers way up and around.

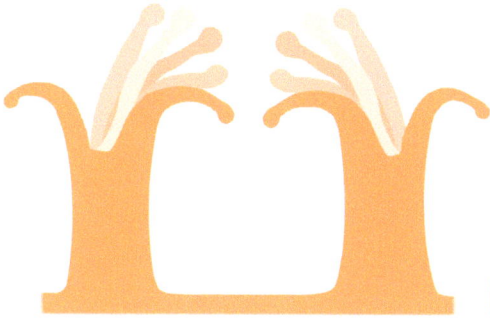

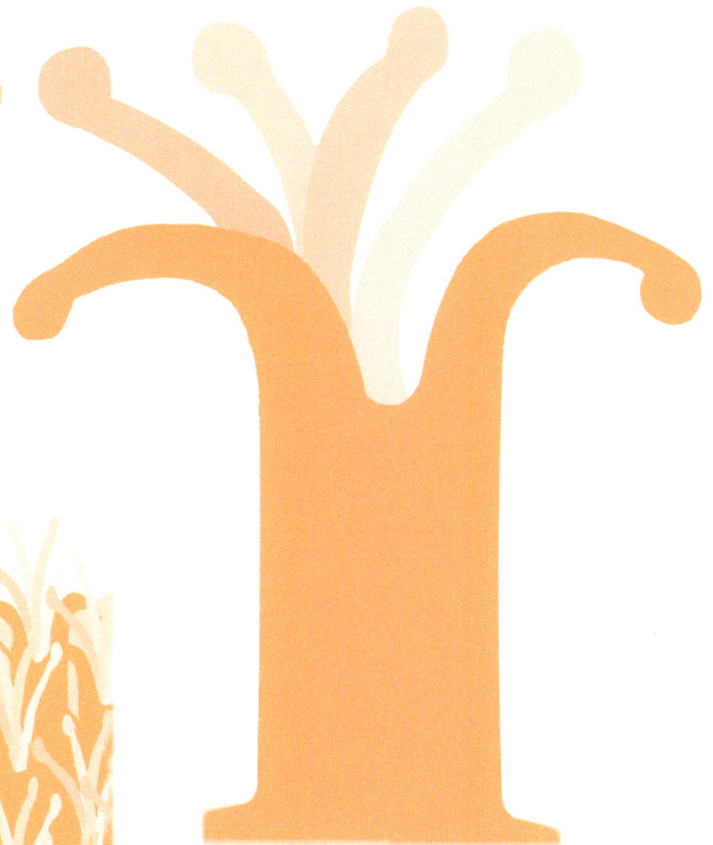

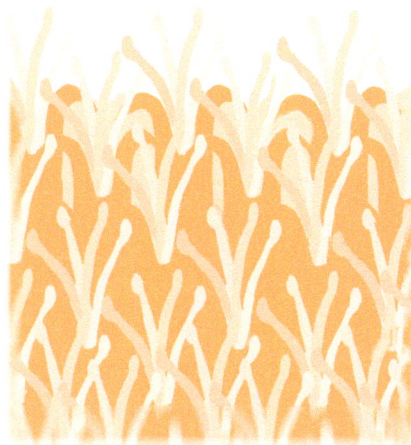

4

The **jelly fish** propels itself by folding and opening itself like an umbrella.

Fold yourself by pushing your middle in with your hands.

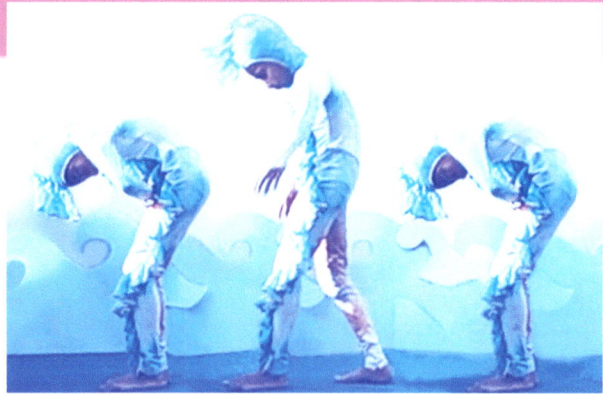

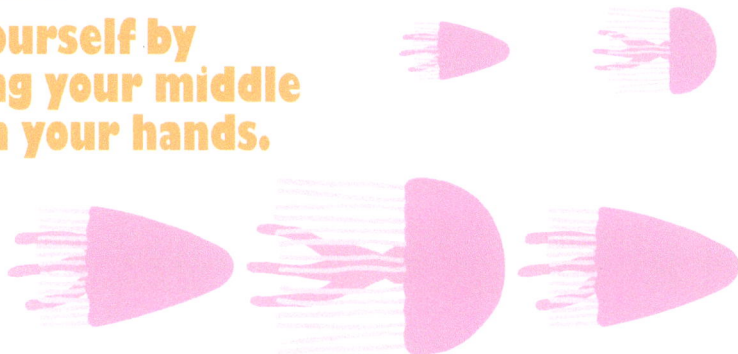

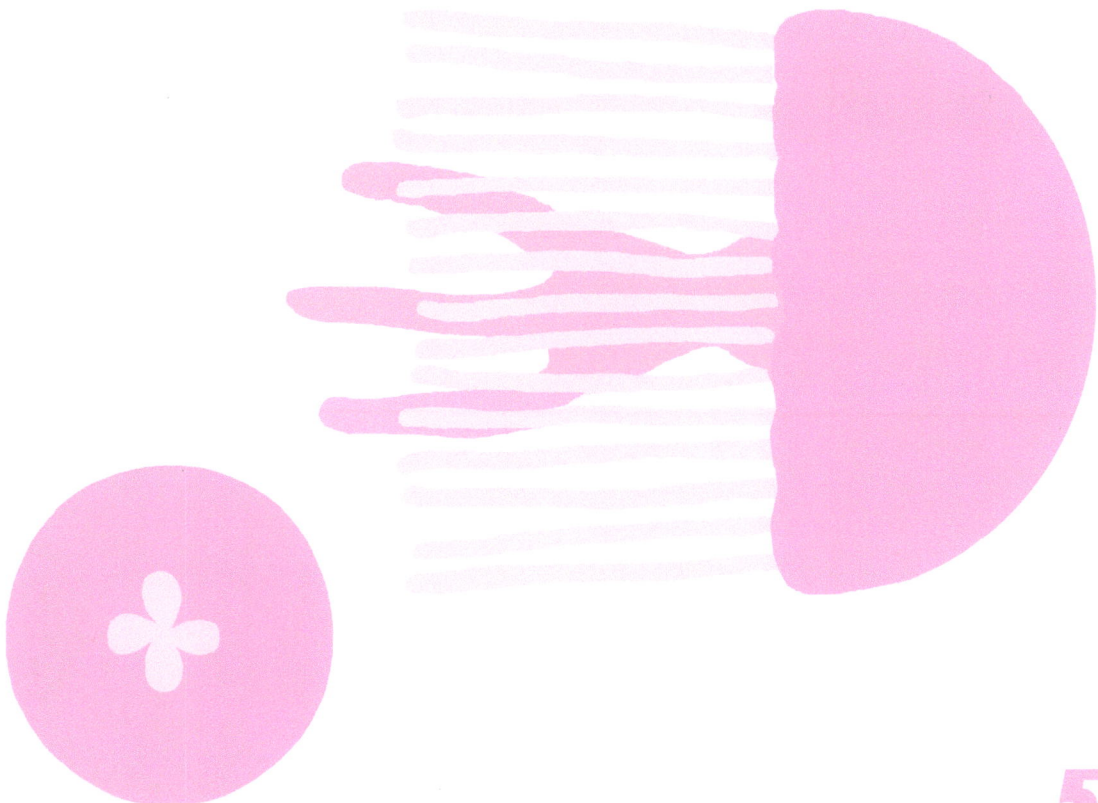

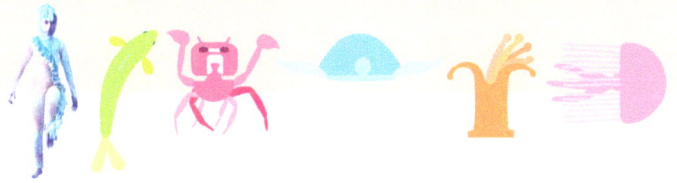

Now you can use these pictures to help you combine the sea animals' movements into a dance.

Between each movement, stand still and do a stampy-stamp movement like you see in the pictures.

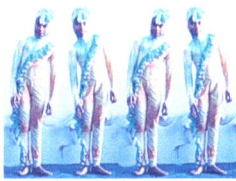

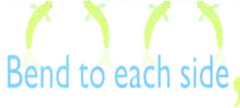

Bend to each side,

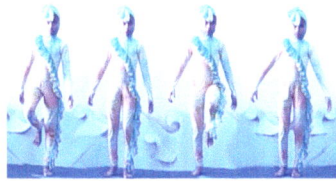

Stampy-stamp-4 times,

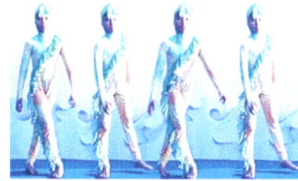

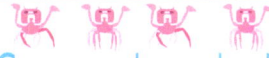

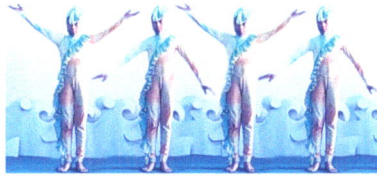

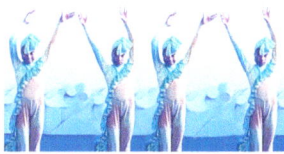

Cross one leg and walk sideways,

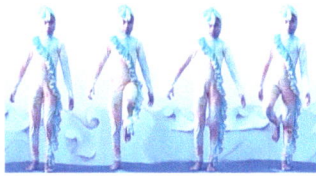

Stampy-stamp-4 times,

Palms up, push air up, turn palms down, push air down,

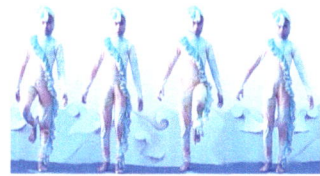

Stampy-stamp-4 times,

On your knees, reach very high, make circles,

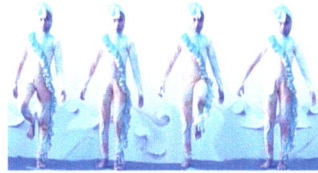

Rise up, Stampy-stamp-4 times,

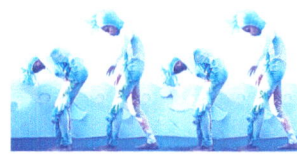

Turn. Push your belly in to fold, let go, and step back,

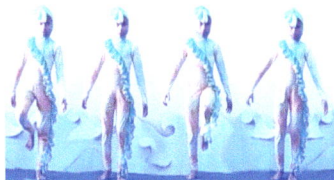

Turn again, to the front. Stampy stamp-4 times, and you're done ☺

6

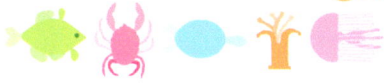

How would this fantasy sea animal move?
Can you do its wiggle?

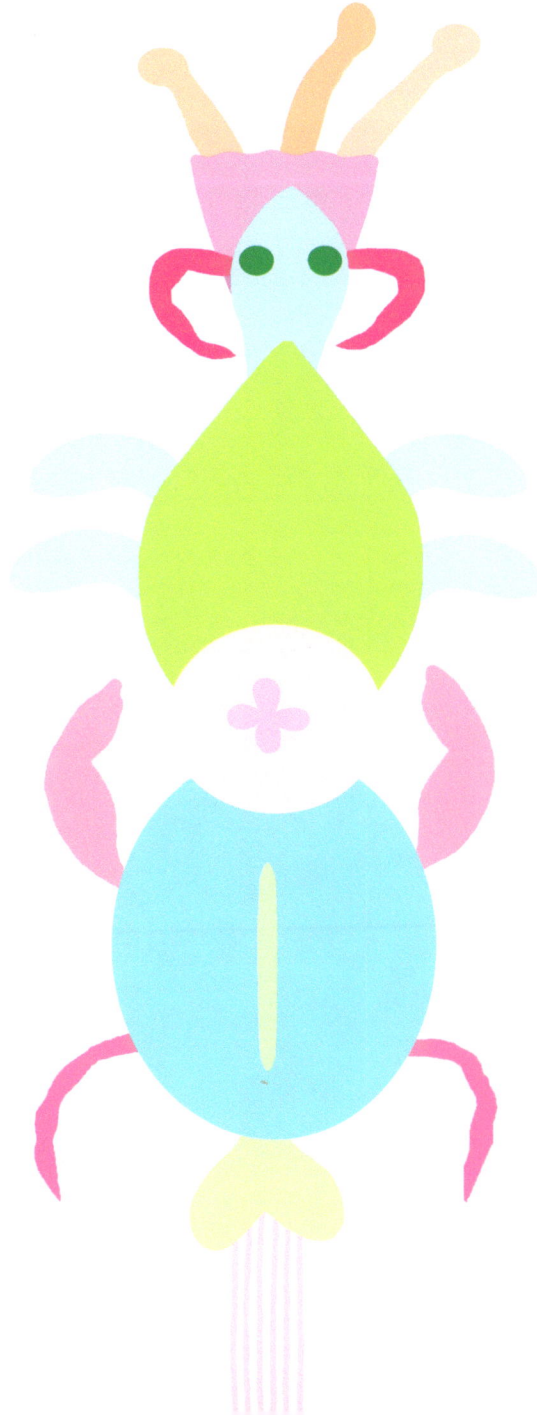

Now create **your own** fantasy sea animal.
Cut these parts out and paste them together
on the next page.

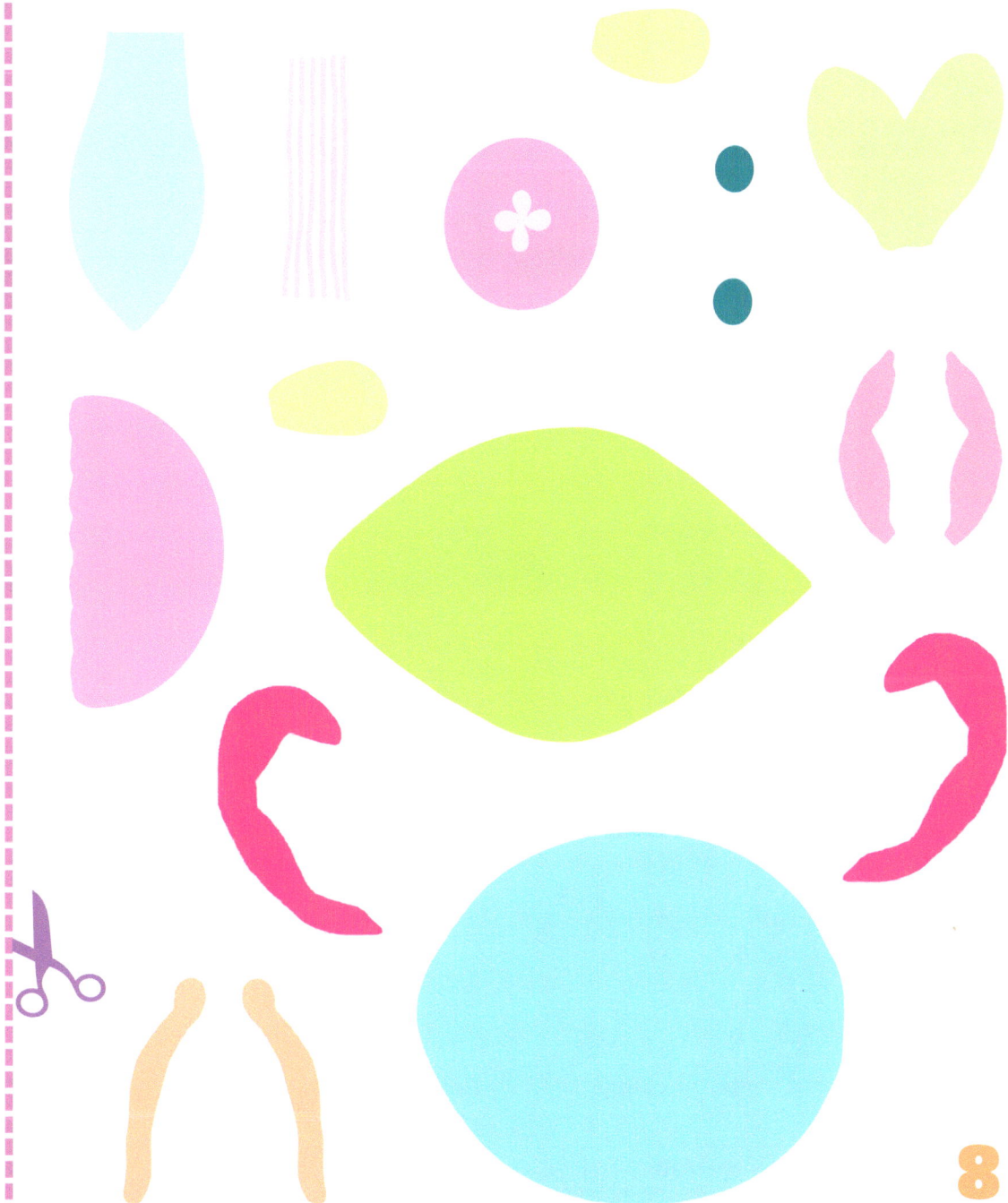

8

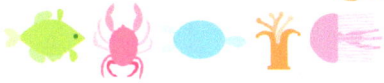

Paste **your** fantasy sea animal here and then make up your own wiggle dance for it.

Bend your body from side-to-side like a fish, and walk in a straight line.

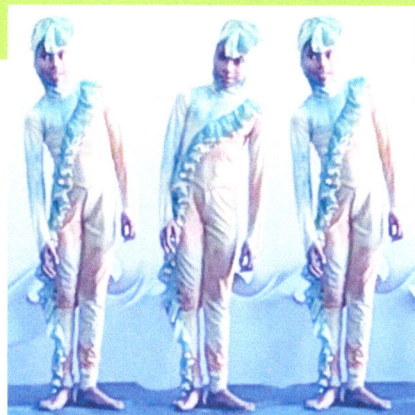

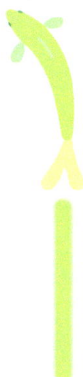

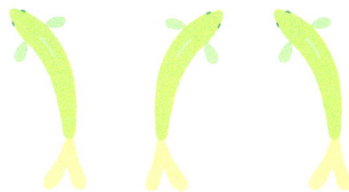

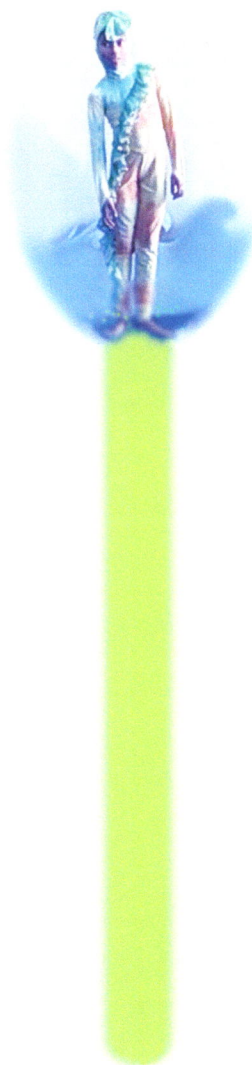

10

Cross one leg in front of the other, like a **crab,** and walk sideways on a round path.

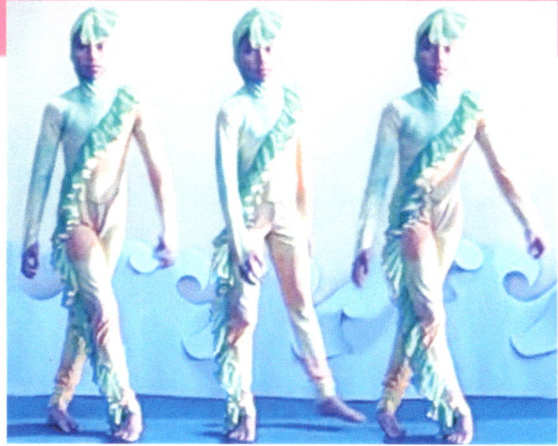

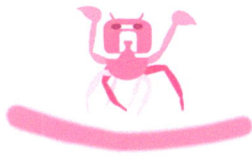

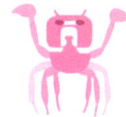

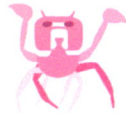

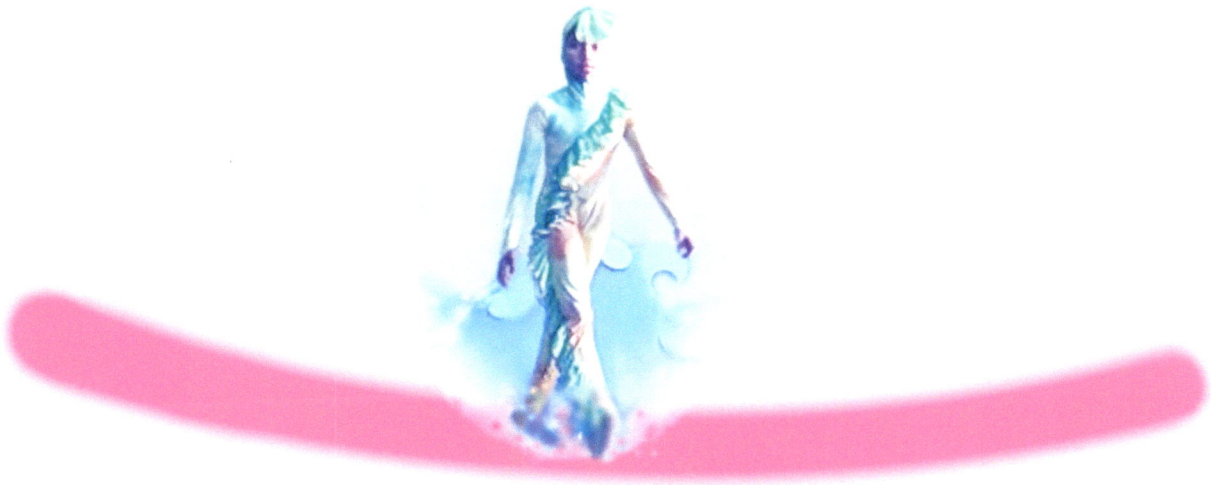

Like a **turtle**, move your arms up and down in a figure eight, and travel along a wavy path.

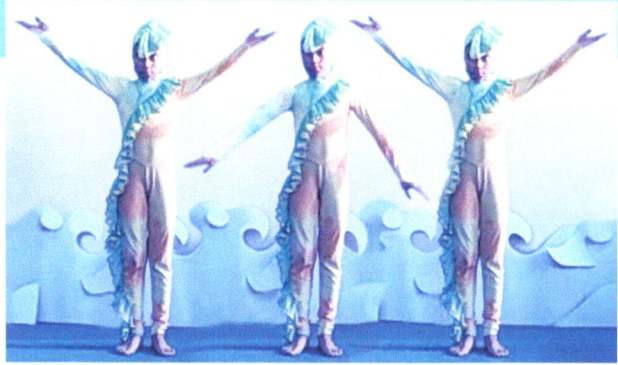

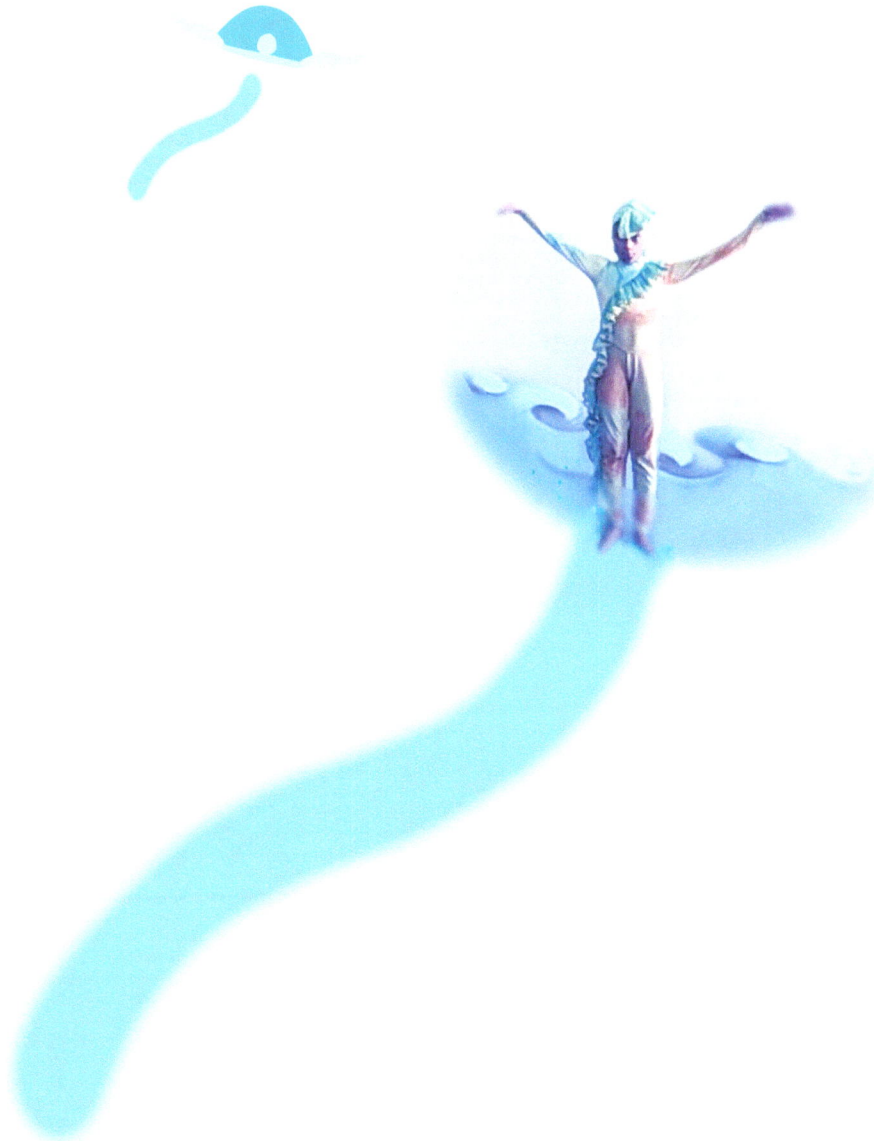

12

Imagine you are under water and have many tentacles, like **coral polyps** do.

Wave your arms high, around and around and around.

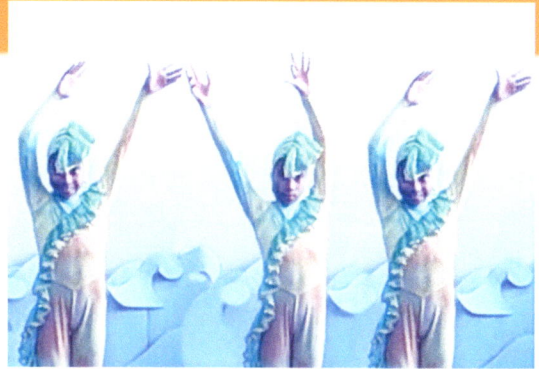

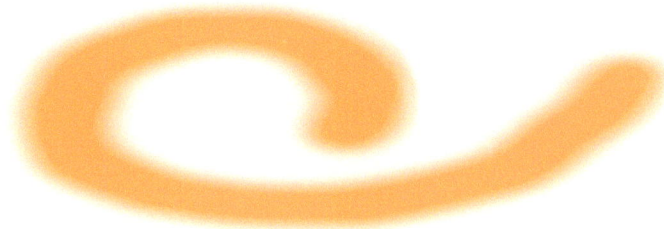

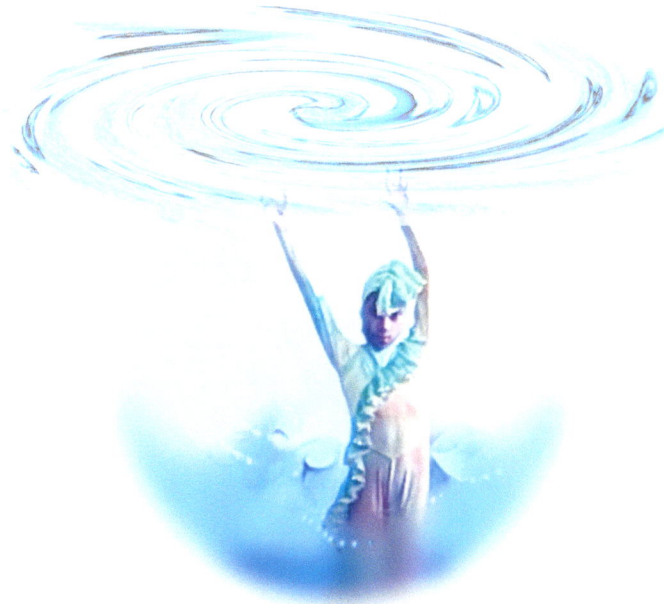

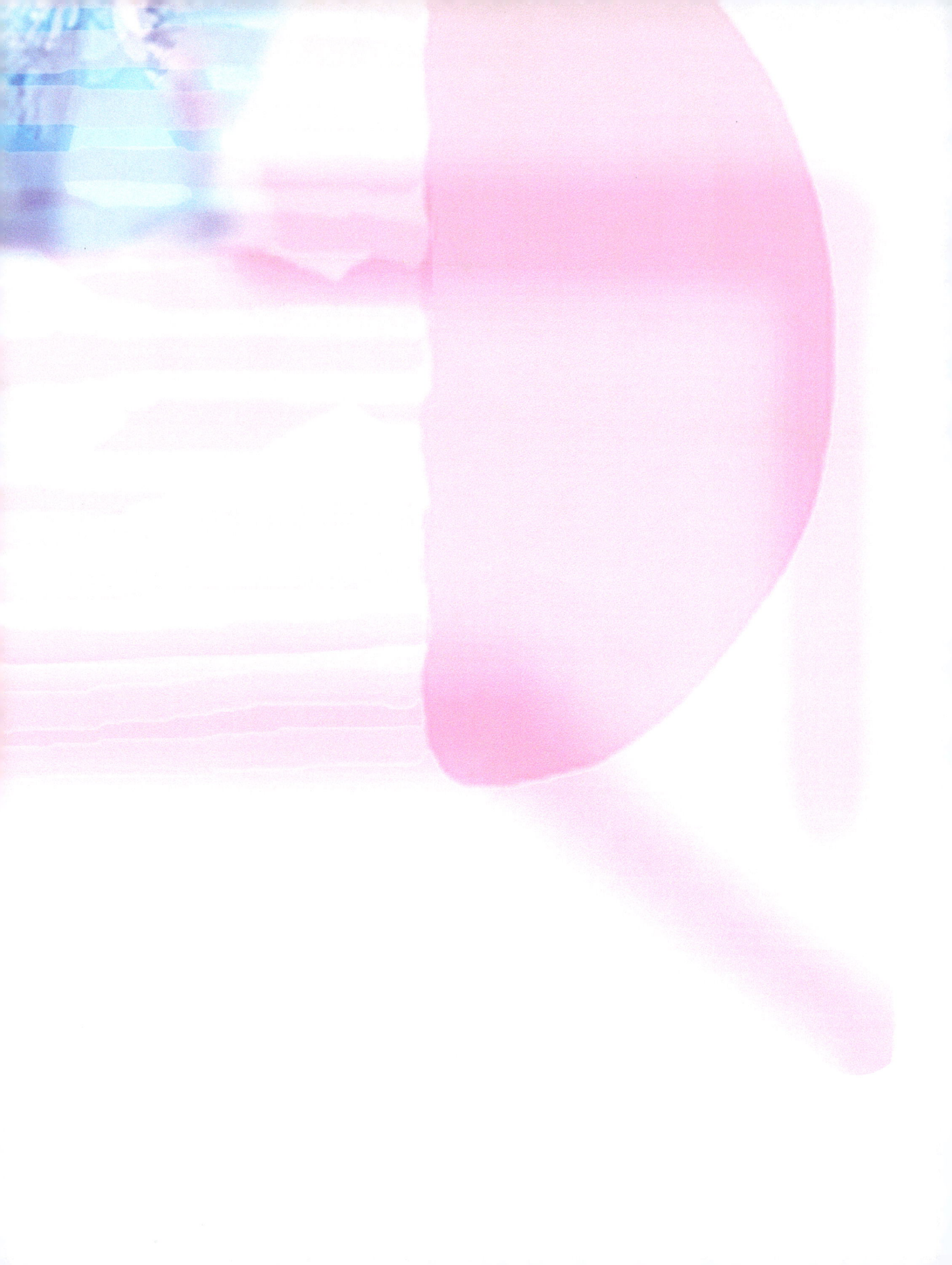

Fold and unfold like an umbrella and go like a jelly fish on the path that you wish.

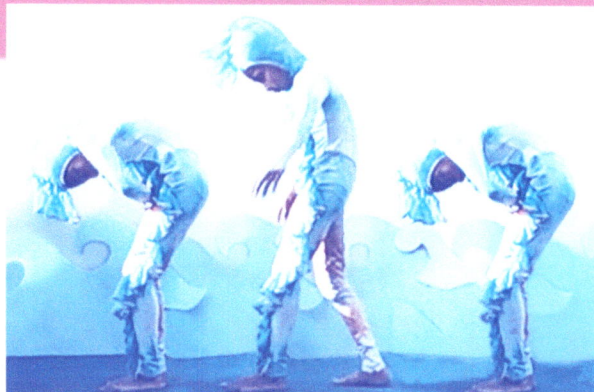

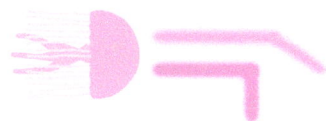

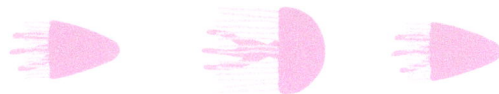

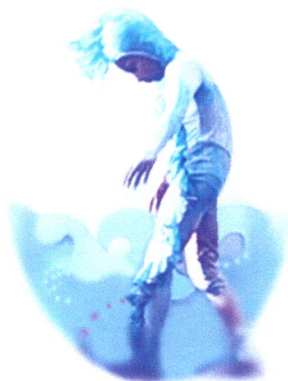

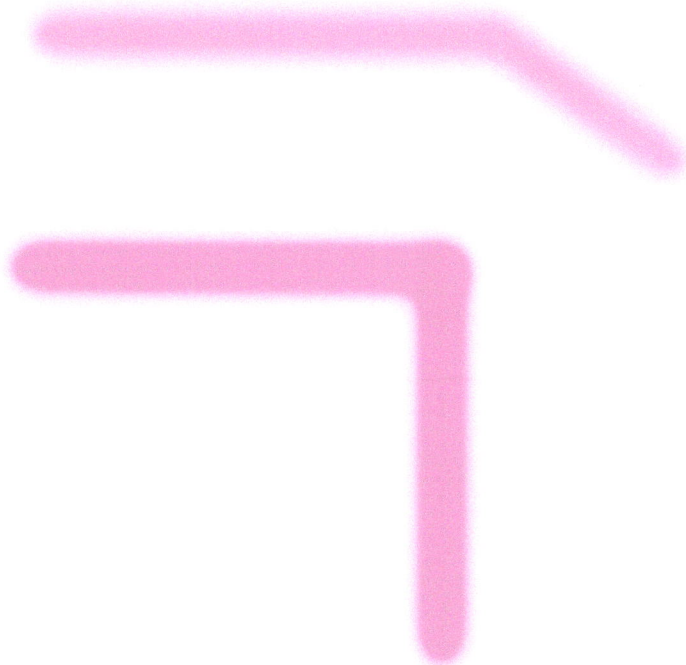

14

...•...paste..write...draw..**Wiggle** some more...and draw...paste...

...and draw...write...paste..wiggle...and draw..paste..write....

...·...paste..write...draw..Wiggle some more...and draw...paste...

...and draw...write...paste...wiggle...and draw...paste...write.....

. . . . . .paste. . .write. . .draw. . .**Wiggle** some more. . .and draw. . .paste. . .

www.ingramcontent.com/pod-product-compliance
Lightning Source LLC
Chambersburg PA
CBHW060833270326
41933CB00002B/77